PEGAN DIET COOKBOOK

Delicious and Nutritious Recipes for a Paleo-Vegan Hybrid Diet

Dr Lily Morgan

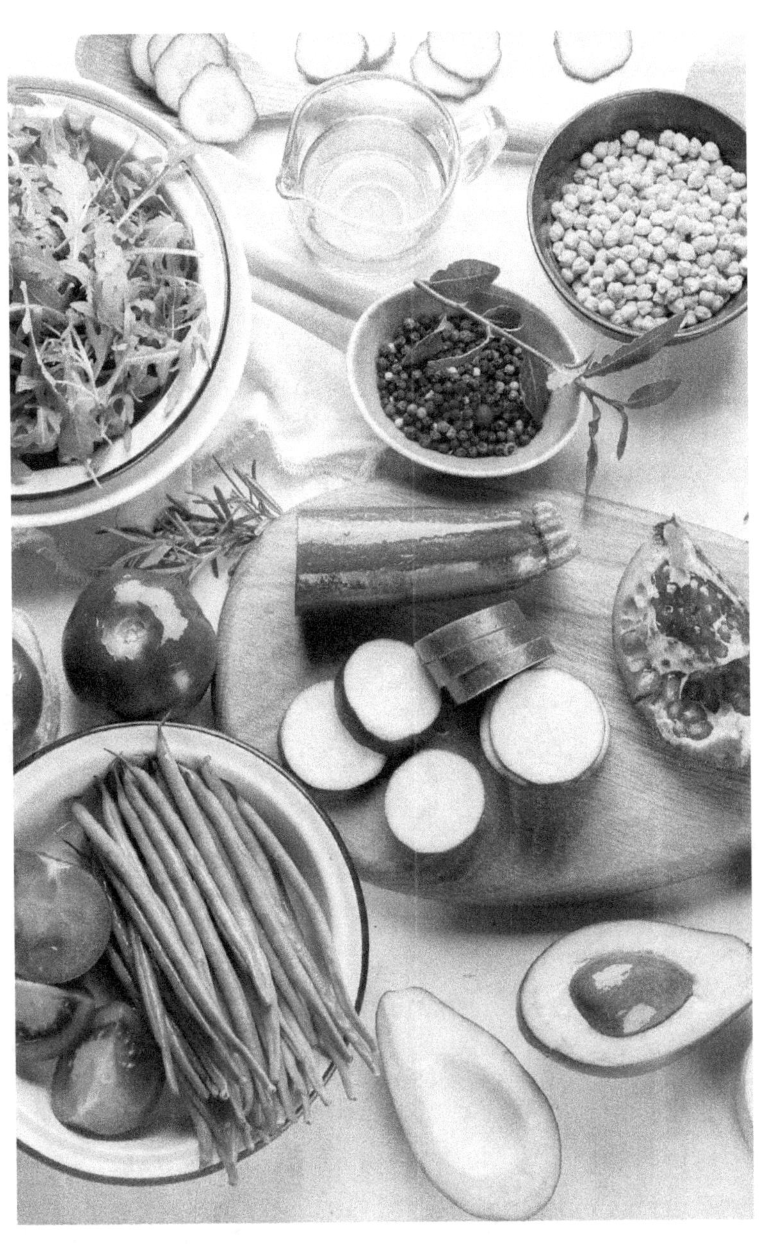

TABLE OF CONTENTS

Chapter 3: Lunch Recipes 37

Chapter 4: Dinner Recipes 54

Chapter 5: Snacks and Appetizers 73

INTRODUCTION

The Pegan Diet is a nutritional approach that combines principles from two popular dietary lifestyles: Paleo and Vegan. This unique fusion seeks to strike a balance between the meat-focused Paleo diet and the plant-based Vegan diet, aiming to provide a more holistic and sustainable way of eating.

Here are some key aspects of the Pegan Diet:

Emphasis on Whole Foods: The Pegan Diet encourages the consumption of whole, unprocessed foods. This means opting for fresh fruits, vegetables, nuts, seeds, and lean proteins rather than heavily processed and refined items.

Plant-Centric: Plants take center stage in the Pegan Diet. A significant portion of your plate should consist of colorful vegetables, both cooked and raw, ensuring a rich intake of vitamins, minerals, and fiber.

Quality Protein Sources: While it leans towards a plant-based approach, the Pegan Diet allows for high-quality protein sources like grass-fed meat, wild-caught fish, and pastured eggs. These provide essential amino acids and nutrients.

Healthy Fats: Good fats are promoted in this diet, such as avocados, nuts, seeds, and olive oil. These fats support overall health, including heart health and brain function.

Low in Sugar: The Pegan Diet is generally low in added sugars. It discourages sugary snacks, desserts, and beverages that can lead to energy spikes and crashes.

Avoidance of Processed Foods: Highly processed foods, including refined grains, artificial additives, and preservatives, are discouraged. The focus is on eating foods in their most natural state.

Benefits of the Pegan Diet:

1. **Nutrient-Dense**: By incorporating a wide variety of fruits, vegetables, and quality proteins, the Pegan

Diet provides a broad spectrum of essential nutrients, supporting overall health.

2. **Weight Management:** The diet's emphasis on whole foods and reduced sugar intake may help with weight management and weight loss goals.

3. **Balanced Blood Sugar:** The Pegan Diet can contribute to stable blood sugar levels due to its low glycemic index foods and emphasis on fiber-rich options.

4. **Heart Health:** Healthy fats and reduced intake of processed foods can support heart health by improving cholesterol profiles and reducing the risk of cardiovascular diseases.

5. **Gut Health:** The abundance of fiber-rich foods can promote a healthy gut microbiome, which is crucial for digestion and immune function.

6. **Sustainability**: By encouraging the consumption of locally sourced, seasonal, and organic foods, the Pegan Diet promotes sustainable eating practices that are good for the planet.

Remember, the Pegan Diet isn't a one-size-fits-all solution, and individual needs may vary. It's essential to consult with a healthcare provider or nutritionist before making significant dietary changes to ensure they align with your specific health goals and requirements.

Chapter 1: 30 Day Meal Plan

Week 1

Day 1:

- Breakfast: Pegan Power Breakfast Bowl
- Lunch: Pegan Mediterranean Salad
- Dinner: Lemon Garlic Herb Grilled Chicken
- Snacks: Guacamole with Veggie Sticks
- Dessert: Pegan Chocolate Avocado Mousse

Day 2:

- Breakfast: Almond Flour Pancakes
- Lunch: Spicy Chickpea and Quinoa Bowl
- Dinner: Baked Salmon with Dill Sauce
- Snacks: Roasted Red Pepper Hummus
- Dessert: Mixed Berry Chia Seed Pudding

Day 3:

- Breakfast: Veggie-Packed Omelette
- Lunch: Pesto Zucchini Noodles
- Dinner: Cauliflower Crust Pizza

- Snacks: Pegan Trail Mix
- Dessert: Almond Butter Cups

Day 4:

- Breakfast: Berry and Coconut Chia Pudding
- Lunch: Thai-Inspired Cabbage Wraps
- Dinner: Beef and Broccoli Stir-Fry
- Snacks: Cucumber and Tomato Salsa
- Dessert: Coconut Macaroons

Day 5:

- Breakfast: Avocado and Salmon Toast
- Lunch: Butternut Squash and Lentil Soup
- Dinner: Pegan Spaghetti Squash Alfredo
- Snacks: Spicy Edamame
- Dessert: Pegan Banana Bread

Day 6:

- Breakfast: Green Smoothie Bowl
- Lunch: Grilled Portobello Mushroom Burger
- Dinner: Moroccan-Inspired Chickpea Stew
- Snacks: Almond-Stuffed Dates

- Dessert: Chocolate Dipped Strawberries

Day 7:

- Breakfast: Sweet Potato Hash with Eggs
- Lunch: Roasted Veggie and Quinoa Salad
- Dinner: Stuffed Acorn Squash
- Snacks: Stuffed Mini Peppers
- Dessert: Blueberry Almond Crisp

Week 2

Day 8:

- Breakfast: Banana Nut Breakfast Muffins
- Lunch: Avocado and Chickpea Salad
- Dinner: Lemon Herb Shrimp Skewers
- Snacks: Coconut-Crusted Tofu Bites
- Dessert: Pecan Pie Energy Bites

Day 9:

- Breakfast: Spinach and Mushroom Frittata
- Lunch: Sweet Potato and Black Bean Quesadilla
- Dinner: Turkey and Sweet Potato Chili
- Snacks: Greek Yogurt Dip with Veggies

- Dessert: No-Bake Cashew Cheesecake

Day 10:

- Breakfast: Quinoa Breakfast Porridge
- Lunch: Cucumber and Avocado Sushi Rolls
- Dinner: Pegan Eggplant Parmesan
- Snacks: Avocado and Cilantro Lime Dip
- Dessert: Avocado Chocolate Truffles

Day 11:

- Breakfast: Pegan Blueberry Muffins
- Lunch: Rainbow Veggie Stir-Fry
- Dinner: Ginger Tofu and Broccoli
- Snacks: Zucchini Fritters
- Dessert: Lemon Poppy Seed Muffins

Day 12:

- Breakfast: Zucchini and Egg Breakfast Casserole
- Lunch: Cauliflower and Broccoli Soup
- Dinner: Quinoa-Stuffed Bell Peppers
- Snacks: Roasted Chickpeas
- Dessert: Raspberry Coconut Bars

Day 13:

- Breakfast: Breakfast Burrito Bowl
- Lunch: Pegan Tofu and Veggie Stir-Fry
- Dinner: Creamy Mushroom and Spinach Pasta
- Snacks: Mixed Nut Energy Bars
- Dessert: Apple Cinnamon Oat Cookies

Day 14:

- Breakfast: Pumpkin Spice Smoothie
- Lunch: Kale and Quinoa Salad with Lemon Tahini Dressing
- Dinner: Teriyaki Glazed Tempeh
- Snacks: Pegan Popcorn
- Dessert: Mango Sorbet

Week 3

Day 15:

- Breakfast: Mixed Berry Parfait
- Lunch: Mediterranean Stuffed Bell Peppers
- Dinner: Pesto Zoodle Bowl
- Snacks: Sweet Potato Fries with Chipotle Aioli
- Dessert: Pegan Berry Parfait

Day 16:

- Breakfast: Pegan Power Breakfast Bowl
- Lunch: Pegan Mediterranean Salad
- Dinner: Lemon Garlic Herb Grilled Chicken
- Snacks: Guacamole with Veggie Sticks
- Dessert: Pegan Chocolate Avocado Mousse

Day 17:

- Breakfast: Almond Flour Pancakes
- Lunch: Spicy Chickpea and Quinoa Bowl
- Dinner: Baked Salmon with Dill Sauce
- Snacks: Roasted Red Pepper Hummus
- Dessert: Mixed Berry Chia Seed Pudding

Day 18:

- Breakfast: Veggie-Packed Omelette
- Lunch: Pesto Zucchini Noodles
- Dinner: Cauliflower Crust Pizza
- Snacks: Pegan Trail Mix
- Dessert: Almond Butter Cups

Day 19:

- Breakfast: Berry and Coconut Chia Pudding
- Lunch: Thai-Inspired Cabbage Wraps
- Dinner: Beef and Broccoli Stir-Fry
- Snacks: Cucumber and Tomato Salsa
- Dessert: Coconut Macaroons

Day 20:

- Breakfast: Avocado and Salmon Toast
- Lunch: Butternut Squash and Lentil Soup
- Dinner: Pegan Spaghetti Squash Alfredo
- Snacks: Spicy Edamame
- Dessert: Pegan Banana Bread

Day 21:

- Breakfast: Green Smoothie Bowl
- Lunch: Grilled Portobello Mushroom Burger
- Dinner: Moroccan-Inspired Chickpea Stew
- Snacks: Almond-Stuffed Dates
- Dessert: Chocolate Dipped Strawberries

Week 4

Day 22:

- Breakfast: Sweet Potato Hash with Eggs
- Lunch: Roasted Veggie and Quinoa Salad
- Dinner: Stuffed Acorn Squash
- Snacks: Stuffed Mini Peppers
- Dessert: Blueberry Almond Crisp

Day 23:

- Breakfast: Banana Nut Breakfast Muffins
- Lunch: Avocado and Chickpea Salad
- Dinner: Lemon Herb Shrimp Skewers
- Snacks: Coconut-Crusted Tofu Bites
- Dessert: Pecan Pie Energy Bites

Day 24:

- Breakfast: Spinach and Mushroom Frittata
- Lunch: Sweet Potato and Black Bean Quesadilla
- Dinner: Turkey and Sweet Potato Chili
- Snacks: Greek Yogurt Dip with Veggies
- Dessert: No-Bake Cashew Cheesecake

Day 25:

- Breakfast: Quinoa Breakfast Porridge
- Lunch: Cucumber and Avocado Sushi Rolls
- Dinner: Pegan Eggplant Parmesan
- Snacks: Avocado and Cilantro Lime Dip
- Dessert: Avocado Chocolate Truffles

Day 26:

- Breakfast: Zucchini and Egg Breakfast Casserole
- Lunch: Cauliflower and Broccoli Soup
- Dinner: Quinoa-Stuffed Bell Peppers
- Snacks: Roasted Chickpeas
- Dessert: Raspberry Coconut Bars

Day 27:

- Breakfast: Breakfast Burrito Bowl
- Lunch: Pegan Tofu and Veggie Stir-Fry
- Dinner: Creamy Mushroom and Spinach Pasta
- Snacks: Mixed Nut Energy Bars
- Dessert: Apple Cinnamon Oat Cookies

Day 28:

- Breakfast: Pumpkin Spice Smoothie
- Lunch: Kale and Quinoa Salad with Lemon Tahini Dressing
- Dinner: Teriyaki Glazed Tempeh
- Snacks: Pegan Popcorn
- Dessert: Mango Sorbet

Day 29:

- Breakfast: Mixed Berry Parfait
- Lunch: Mediterranean Stuffed Bell Peppers
- Dinner: Pesto Zoodle Bowl
- Snacks: Sweet Potato Fries with Chipotle Aioli
- Dessert: Pegan Berry Parfait

Day 30:

- Breakfast: Pegan Power Breakfast Bowl
- Lunch: Pegan Mediterranean Salad
- Dinner: Lemon Garlic Herb Grilled Chicken
- Snacks: Guacamole with Veggie Sticks
- Dessert: Pegan Chocolate Avocado Mousse

Congratulations on completing your 30-day Pegan diet journey! You've enjoyed a variety of delicious and nutritious meals.

Chapter 2: Breakfast Recipes

Welcome to the delightful world of morning nourishment in our "Pegan Diet Cookbook." Here in Chapter 2, we'll take you on a journey through nutritious and energizing breakfast recipes that will kickstart your day on a healthy note. From hearty bowls to fluffy pancakes, we've got your breakfast cravings covered.

Pegan Power Breakfast Bowl

Ingredients:

- 1/2 cup cooked quinoa
- 1/4 cup mixed berries
- 1 tablespoon almond butter
- 1 tablespoon chopped nuts
- 1 teaspoon honey (optional)

Instructions:

1. In a bowl, layer the cooked quinoa.
2. Top it with mixed berries, almond butter, chopped nuts, and a drizzle of honey if desired.

3. Mix everything together and enjoy your power-
   packed breakfast.

Almond Flour Pancakes

Ingredients:

- 1 cup almond flour
- 2 eggs
- 1/4 cup almond milk
- 1 teaspoon baking powder
- 1/2 teaspoon vanilla extract

Instructions:

1. In a bowl, whisk together almond flour, eggs, almond milk, baking powder, and vanilla extract until you have a smooth batter.
2. Heat a non-stick skillet over medium heat and ladle in the pancake batter.
3. Cook until bubbles form on the surface, then flip and cook until golden brown.
4. Serve with your favorite Pegan-friendly toppings.

Veggie-Packed Omelette

Ingredients:

- 2 eggs
- 1/4 cup diced bell peppers
- 1/4 cup diced tomatoes
- 1/4 cup diced spinach
- Salt and pepper to taste

Instructions:

1. Whisk the eggs in a bowl and season with salt and pepper.
2. Heat a skillet over medium-high heat and add a touch of olive oil.
3. Pour in the whisked eggs and sprinkle diced vegetables on top.
4. Cook until the eggs set, then fold the omelette in half.
5. Slide it onto a plate and enjoy your veggie-packed delight.

Berry and Coconut Chia Pudding

Ingredients:

- 2 tablespoons chia seeds
- 1/2 cup coconut milk
- 1/4 cup mixed berries
- 1 teaspoon honey (optional)

Instructions:

1. In a jar, mix chia seeds and coconut milk.
2. Let it sit in the refrigerator for a few hours or overnight to thicken.
3. Top with mixed berries and a drizzle of honey if desired.
4. Stir, and your delightful chia pudding is ready to enjoy.

Avocado and Salmon Toast

Ingredients:

- 1 slice of Pegan-friendly bread
- 1/2 ripe avocado, mashed
- Smoked salmon slices

- Lemon juice and zest
- Fresh dill

Instructions:

1. Toast the bread to your desired level of crispiness.
2. Spread mashed avocado on the toast.
3. Layer smoked salmon on top.
4. Sprinkle with lemon zest, a squeeze of lemon juice, and fresh dill.
5. Savor the flavors of this elegant toast.

Green Smoothie Bowl

Ingredients:

- 1 cup spinach
- 1/2 banana
- 1/2 cup unsweetened almond milk
- 1 tablespoon chia seeds
- Toppings: sliced banana, granola, and berries

Instructions:

1. Blend spinach, banana, and almond milk until smooth.

2. Pour the green smoothie into a bowl.

3. Top with chia seeds, sliced banana, granola, and a handful of berries.

4. This vibrant bowl is a refreshing way to start your day.

Sweet Potato Hash with Eggs

Ingredients:

- 1 sweet potato, diced
- 1/4 cup diced bell peppers
- 1/4 cup diced onions
- 2 eggs
- Olive oil
- Paprika and salt to taste

Instructions:

1. Heat olive oil in a skillet over medium heat.

2. Add sweet potato, bell peppers, and onions. Season with paprika and salt.

3. Cook until sweet potatoes are tender and slightly crispy.

4. Make two wells in the hash and crack eggs into them.

5. Cover and cook until the eggs are done to your liking.

6. Serve your hearty sweet potato hash with perfectly cooked eggs.

Banana Nut Breakfast Muffins

Ingredients:

- 2 ripe bananas, mashed
- 2 eggs
- 1/4 cup almond flour
- 1/4 cup chopped nuts (e.g., walnuts or pecans)
- 1 teaspoon baking soda
- Cinnamon and honey (optional)

Instructions:

1. Preheat your oven to 350°F (175°C) and line a muffin tin with liners.

2. In a bowl, mix mashed bananas, eggs, almond flour, chopped nuts, and baking soda.

3. Divide the batter evenly among the muffin cups.

4. Bake for 15-20 minutes or until a toothpick comes out clean.

5. Optionally, drizzle with honey and sprinkle with cinnamon for extra flavor.

Spinach and Mushroom Frittata

Ingredients:

- 6 eggs
- 1 cup spinach, chopped
- 1/2 cup sliced mushrooms
- 1/4 cup diced onions
- Salt and pepper to taste

Instructions:

1. Preheat your oven to 350°F (175°C).
2. In an oven-safe skillet, sauté onions and mushrooms until soft.
3. Add spinach and cook until wilted.
4. Whisk eggs, season with salt and pepper, and pour them over the veggies.
5. Cook on the stovetop for a few minutes, then transfer to the oven and bake until set.
6. Slice into wedges and serve this nutritious frittata.

Quinoa Breakfast Porridge

Ingredients:

- 1/2 cup cooked quinoa
- 1/2 cup almond milk
- 1/4 cup chopped nuts
- 1/4 cup diced dried fruits (e.g., apricots or cranberries)
- Honey or maple syrup (optional)

Instructions:

1. In a saucepan, combine cooked quinoa and almond milk.
2. Heat over medium heat until warm.
3. Stir in chopped nuts and dried fruits.
4. Sweeten with honey or maple syrup if desired.
5. Enjoy a warm and hearty quinoa porridge.

Pegan Blueberry Muffins

Ingredients:

- 1 cup almond flour
- 1/4 cup coconut flour

- 1/2 teaspoon baking soda
- 2 eggs
- 1/4 cup almond milk
- 1/4 cup honey
- 1/2 cup fresh blueberries

Instructions:

1. Preheat your oven to 350°F (175°C) and line a muffin tin with liners.
2. In a bowl, mix almond flour, coconut flour, and baking soda.
3. In a separate bowl, whisk eggs, almond milk, and honey.
4. Combine wet and dry ingredients, then gently fold in blueberries.
5. Spoon the batter into the muffin cups and bake for 20-25 minutes until golden.

Zucchini and Egg Breakfast Casserole

Ingredients:

- 2 zucchinis, grated
- 6 eggs
- 1/2 cup diced tomatoes
- 1/4 cup diced onions
- 1/4 cup chopped fresh basil
- Salt and pepper to taste

Instructions:

1. Preheat your oven to 350°F (175°C).
2. In a bowl, whisk eggs and season with salt and pepper.
3. Stir in grated zucchini, diced tomatoes, onions, and fresh basil.
4. Pour the mixture into a greased baking dish and bake for 25-30 minutes until set.
5. Slice into squares and serve this savory casserole.

Breakfast Burrito Bowl

Ingredients:

- 2 eggs
- 1/4 cup black beans, drained and rinsed
- 1/4 cup diced bell peppers
- 1/4 cup diced tomatoes
- Sliced avocado
- Salsa

Instructions:

1. Scramble the eggs in a pan over medium heat.
2. In a bowl, layer scrambled eggs, black beans, diced bell peppers, diced tomatoes, and sliced avocado.
3. Top with your favorite salsa for a burst of flavor.

Pumpkin Spice Smoothie

Ingredients:

- 1/2 cup pumpkin puree
- 1 banana
- 1/2 cup almond milk
- 1/2 teaspoon pumpkin spice

- 1 tablespoon honey (optional)

Instructions:

1. Blend pumpkin puree, banana, almond milk, pumpkin spice, and honey until smooth.
2. Pour into a glass and enjoy the warm flavors of fall.

Mixed Berry Parfait

Ingredients:

- 1 cup mixed berries (e.g., strawberries, blueberries, raspberries)
- 1 cup Greek yogurt
- 1/4 cup granola

Instructions:

1. In a glass or bowl, layer mixed berries, Greek yogurt, and granola.
2. Repeat the layers.
3. Finish with a sprinkle of granola on top for added crunch.

Chapter 3: Lunch Recipes

Lunchtime is a perfect opportunity to embrace the Pegan way of eating with these delicious and nutritious lunch recipes. Packed with wholesome ingredients, these meals are designed to keep you energized throughout your day.

Pegan Mediterranean Salad

Ingredients:

- 2 cups of mixed greens
- 1/2 cup cherry tomatoes, halved
- 1/4 cup cucumber, diced
- 1/4 cup Kalamata olives, pitted
- 1/4 cup red onion, thinly sliced
- 1/4 cup crumbled feta cheese
- 2 tablespoons extra-virgin olive oil
- 1 tablespoon balsamic vinegar
- Salt and pepper to taste

Instructions:

1. In a large bowl, combine the mixed greens, cherry tomatoes, cucumber, Kalamata olives, red onion, and feta cheese.
2. Drizzle with olive oil and balsamic vinegar. Toss to combine.
3. Season with salt and pepper to taste.
4. Serve and enjoy your Mediterranean-inspired salad.

Spicy Chickpea and Quinoa Bowl

Ingredients:

- 1 cup cooked quinoa
- 1 can (15 oz) chickpeas, drained and rinsed
- 1 tablespoon olive oil
- 1 teaspoon smoked paprika
- 1/2 teaspoon cayenne pepper (adjust to taste)
- Salt and pepper to taste
- 1/2 cup diced bell peppers
- 1/2 cup diced cucumber
- 1/4 cup chopped fresh cilantro
- Juice of 1 lemon

Instructions:

1. Heat olive oil in a skillet over medium heat. Add chickpeas, smoked paprika, cayenne pepper, salt, and pepper. Sauté for 5-7 minutes until chickpeas are crispy.
2. In a bowl, combine cooked quinoa, crispy chickpeas, diced bell peppers, cucumber, and cilantro.
3. Drizzle with lemon juice and toss to mix.
4. Serve your spicy chickpea and quinoa bowl with a burst of flavors.

Pesto Zucchini Noodles

Ingredients:

- 2 large zucchinis, spiralized into noodles
- 1/2 cup cherry tomatoes, halved
- 2 tablespoons pesto sauce
- 1/4 cup pine nuts
- Grated Parmesan cheese (optional)
- Salt and pepper to taste

Instructions:

1. In a large pan, sauté zucchini noodles over medium heat for 2-3 minutes until slightly softened.
2. Toss in cherry tomatoes and pesto sauce, stirring for an additional 2 minutes.
3. Season with salt and pepper to taste.
4. Serve with a sprinkle of pine nuts and optional grated Parmesan cheese.

Thai-Inspired Cabbage Wraps

Ingredients:

*   8 large cabbage leaves, blanched and cooled
*   1 cup cooked quinoa
*   1 cup cooked and shredded chicken (or tofu for a vegetarian option)
*   1/2 cup shredded carrots
*   1/4 cup fresh cilantro leaves
*   1/4 cup chopped peanuts
*   Thai-inspired sauce (mix 3 tablespoons peanut butter, 2 tablespoons soy sauce, 1 tablespoon honey, and 1 teaspoon sriracha)

Instructions:

1. Lay out cabbage leaves.

2. Fill each leaf with quinoa, chicken or tofu, shredded carrots, cilantro leaves, and chopped peanuts.

3. Drizzle with the Thai-inspired sauce.

4. Roll up the cabbage leaves, tucking in the sides.

5. Serve your Thai-inspired cabbage wraps and savor the flavors.

Butternut Squash and Lentil Soup

Ingredients:

- 1 small butternut squash, peeled and diced
- 1 cup red lentils, rinsed and drained
- 1 onion, chopped
- 2 cloves garlic, minced
- 1 teaspoon ground cumin
- 1 teaspoon ground coriander
- 6 cups vegetable broth
- Salt and pepper to taste
- Fresh parsley for garnish

Instructions:

1. In a large pot, sauté the chopped onion and garlic until fragrant.
2. Add the diced butternut squash, red lentils, ground cumin, and ground coriander. Stir for a few minutes.
3. Pour in the vegetable broth and bring to a boil.
4. Reduce the heat, cover, and simmer for about 20-25 minutes until the squash and lentils are tender.
5. Season with salt and pepper to taste.
6. Garnish with fresh parsley before serving.

Grilled Portobello Mushroom Burger

Ingredients:

- 4 large Portobello mushroom caps
- 4 whole-grain burger buns
- 1/4 cup balsamic vinegar
- 2 tablespoons olive oil
- 2 cloves garlic, minced
- 1 teaspoon dried thyme
- Salt and pepper to taste
- Your choice of burger toppings (lettuce, tomato, onion, etc.)

Instructions:

1. In a bowl, whisk together balsamic vinegar, olive oil, minced garlic, dried thyme, salt, and pepper.
2. Brush the Portobello mushroom caps with this marinade.
3. Preheat your grill to medium-high heat.
4. Grill the Portobello mushrooms for about 4-5 minutes per side until tender.
5. Toast the whole-grain burger buns on the grill for a minute or so.
6. Assemble your grilled Portobello mushroom burgers with your favorite toppings.

Roasted Veggie and Quinoa Salad

Ingredients:

- 1 cup cooked quinoa
- 2 cups mixed roasted vegetables (bell peppers, zucchini, cherry tomatoes, etc.)
- 1/4 cup crumbled feta cheese
- 2 tablespoons balsamic vinegar
- 2 tablespoons olive oil
- Fresh basil leaves for garnish

- Salt and pepper to taste

Instructions:

1. In a large bowl, combine cooked quinoa, roasted vegetables, and crumbled feta cheese.
2. Whisk together balsamic vinegar, olive oil, salt, and pepper.
3. Drizzle the dressing over the salad and toss to combine.
4. Garnish with fresh basil leaves before serving.

Avocado and Chickpea Salad

Ingredients:

- 2 ripe avocados, diced
- 1 can (15 oz) chickpeas, drained and rinsed
- 1/4 cup red onion, finely chopped
- 1/4 cup fresh cilantro, chopped
- Juice of 1 lime
- Salt and pepper to taste

Instructions:

1. In a bowl, combine diced avocados, chickpeas, red onion, and fresh cilantro.
2. Drizzle with lime juice and season with salt and pepper.
3. Gently toss to mix.
4. Serve your avocado and chickpea salad as a delicious and satisfying lunch option.

Sweet Potato and Black Bean Quesadilla

Ingredients:

- 2 medium sweet potatoes, peeled and diced
- 1 can (15 oz) black beans, drained and rinsed
- 1 teaspoon ground cumin
- 1/2 teaspoon chili powder
- 4 whole-grain tortillas
- 1 cup shredded dairy-free cheese (optional)
- Guacamole and salsa for serving

Instructions:

1. Steam or boil the diced sweet potatoes until tender. Mash them and set aside.

2. In a separate bowl, mix the black beans with ground cumin and chili powder.

3. Lay out a tortilla and spread mashed sweet potatoes on one half.

4. Add a layer of the seasoned black beans and sprinkle with shredded cheese if desired.

5. Fold the tortilla in half to create a quesadilla.

6. Heat a non-stick skillet over medium heat and cook the quesadilla for 2-3 minutes per side until crispy.

7. Serve with guacamole and salsa.

Cucumber and Avocado Sushi Rolls

Ingredients:

- 2 nori seaweed sheets
- 1 cup sushi rice, cooked and seasoned with rice vinegar
- 1 small cucumber, julienned
- 1 ripe avocado, sliced
- Soy sauce and wasabi for dipping

Instructions:

1. Place a bamboo sushi rolling mat on a clean surface.
2. Lay a sheet of plastic wrap on top of the mat.
3. Place a nori sheet, shiny side down, on the plastic wrap.
4. Spread a layer of sushi rice evenly over the nori, leaving a small border at the top.
5. Arrange cucumber and avocado slices in the center of the rice.
6. Carefully roll up the sushi using the bamboo mat, applying gentle pressure.
7. Wet the exposed nori edge with water to seal the roll.
8. Slice the roll into bite-sized pieces with a sharp knife.
9. Serve with soy sauce and wasabi for dipping.

Rainbow Veggie Stir-Fry

Ingredients:

- 2 cups mixed colorful bell peppers, sliced
- 1 cup broccoli florets
- 1 cup snap peas
- 1 cup sliced carrots
- 1 cup sliced mushrooms

- 1/4 cup low-sodium soy sauce or tamari
- 1 tablespoon sesame oil
- 1 tablespoon minced ginger
- 2 cloves garlic, minced
- Cooked brown rice or quinoa for serving

Instructions:

1. Heat sesame oil in a large skillet or wok over medium-high heat.
2. Add minced ginger and garlic, sauté for 30 seconds.
3. Add the sliced vegetables and stir-fry for about 5-7 minutes until tender-crisp.
4. Pour in the soy sauce and stir to coat the veggies evenly.
5. Serve your rainbow veggie stir-fry over cooked brown rice or quinoa.

Cauliflower and Broccoli Soup

Ingredients:

- 1 cauliflower head, chopped
- 2 cups broccoli florets
- 1 onion, chopped

- 2 cloves garlic, minced

- 4 cups vegetable broth

- 1 cup unsweetened almond milk (or other non-dairy milk)

- Salt and pepper to taste

- Fresh chives for garnish (optional)

Instructions:

1. In a large pot, sauté the chopped onion and garlic until translucent.

2. Add the chopped cauliflower, broccoli florets, and vegetable broth to the pot.

3. Bring to a boil, then reduce heat and simmer for 20-25 minutes until vegetables are tender.

4. Use an immersion blender to puree the soup until smooth.

5. Stir in the almond milk and heat through.

6. Season with salt and pepper to taste.

7. Garnish with fresh chives if desired.

Pegan Tofu and Veggie Stir-Fry

Ingredients:

- 1 block extra-firm tofu, cubed
- 2 cups mixed vegetables (bell peppers, broccoli, snap peas, etc.)
- 2 tablespoons low-sodium soy sauce or tamari
- 1 tablespoon sesame oil
- 1 tablespoon rice vinegar
- 1 tablespoon honey or maple syrup
- 1 clove garlic, minced
- 1 teaspoon minced ginger
- Cooked quinoa or brown rice for serving

Instructions:

1. In a small bowl, whisk together soy sauce, sesame oil, rice vinegar, honey or maple syrup, garlic, and ginger to make the sauce.
2. Heat a non-stick skillet over medium-high heat and add cubed tofu. Cook until browned on all sides.
3. Remove tofu from the skillet and set aside.
4. In the same skillet, add mixed vegetables and stir-fry for about 5 minutes until tender-crisp.

5. Return tofu to the skillet, pour the sauce over the tofu and vegetables, and stir to coat.

6. Serve your Pegan tofu and veggie stir-fry over cooked quinoa or brown rice.

Kale and Quinoa Salad with Lemon Tahini Dressing

Ingredients:

- 2 cups cooked quinoa
- 3 cups kale leaves, stems removed and chopped
- 1/4 cup cherry tomatoes, halved
- 1/4 cup diced cucumber
- 1/4 cup diced red bell pepper
- 1/4 cup sliced almonds
- Lemon Tahini Dressing (whisk together 3 tablespoons tahini, juice of 1 lemon, 1 clove garlic, minced, and water to thin)
- Salt and pepper to taste

Instructions:

1. In a large bowl, combine cooked quinoa, chopped kale, cherry tomatoes, cucumber, and red bell pepper.
2. Drizzle with Lemon Tahini Dressing and toss to coat.
3. Sprinkle with sliced almonds for added crunch.
4. Season with salt and pepper to taste.
5. Enjoy your nutritious and flavorful kale and quinoa salad.

Mediterranean Stuffed Bell Peppers

Ingredients:

- 4 bell peppers, any color
- 1 cup cooked quinoa
- 1 can (15 oz) chickpeas, drained and rinsed
- 1/2 cup diced cucumber
- 1/2 cup cherry tomatoes, halved
- 1/4 cup Kalamata olives, pitted and sliced
- 1/4 cup crumbled feta cheese (optional)
- Fresh parsley for garnish
- Olive oil and lemon juice for drizzling
- Salt and pepper to taste

Instructions:

1. Preheat your oven to 375°F (190°C).

2. Cut the tops off the bell peppers and remove the seeds and membranes.

3. In a bowl, combine cooked quinoa, chickpeas, diced cucumber, cherry tomatoes, Kalamata olives, and crumbled feta cheese (if using).

4. Stuff each bell pepper with the quinoa mixture.

5. Place stuffed bell peppers in a baking dish and drizzle with olive oil and lemon juice.

6. Season with salt and pepper.

7. Bake for 30-35 minutes until the peppers are tender.

8. Garnish with fresh parsley before serving.

Chapter 4: Dinner Recipes

In this chapter, we embark on a culinary journey through delicious and wholesome dinner recipes, each carefully crafted to align with the principles of the Pegan diet. From succulent meats to hearty vegetarian options, these recipes will satisfy your cravings while keeping you on the path to better health.

Lemon Garlic Herb Grilled Chicken

Ingredients:

- 4 boneless, skinless chicken breasts
- 2 tablespoons olive oil
- 2 cloves garlic, minced
- Zest and juice of 1 lemon
- 1 teaspoon dried rosemary
- 1 teaspoon dried thyme
- Salt and pepper to taste

Instructions:

1. In a bowl, whisk together the olive oil, garlic, lemon zest, lemon juice, rosemary, thyme, salt, and pepper.

2. Place the chicken breasts in a resealable plastic bag and pour the marinade over them. Seal the bag and refrigerate for at least 30 minutes.

3. Preheat your grill to medium-high heat. Remove the chicken from the marinade and grill for about 6-8 minutes per side or until fully cooked.

Baked Salmon with Dill Sauce

Ingredients:

- 4 salmon fillets
- 2 tablespoons olive oil
- 2 tablespoons fresh dill, chopped
- 1 lemon, thinly sliced
- Salt and pepper to taste

Instructions:

1. Preheat your oven to 375°F (190°C). Place the salmon fillets on a baking sheet lined with parchment paper.

2. Drizzle the olive oil over the salmon and season with dill, salt, and pepper. Place lemon slices on top of each fillet.

3. Bake for about 15-20 minutes or until the salmon flakes easily with a fork.

Cauliflower Crust Pizza

Ingredients:

- 1 medium cauliflower head, florets only
- 1 egg
- 1 cup shredded mozzarella cheese
- 1/2 teaspoon dried oregano
- 1/2 teaspoon garlic powder
- Pizza sauce and toppings of your choice

Instructions:

1. Preheat your oven to 450°F (230°C). Place cauliflower florets in a food processor and pulse until they resemble rice.

2. Microwave the cauliflower rice for 4-5 minutes, then let it cool. Squeeze out excess moisture using a clean kitchen towel.

3. In a bowl, combine the cauliflower rice, egg, mozzarella cheese, oregano, and garlic powder.

4. Press the mixture onto a parchment-lined baking sheet to form a crust. Bake for about 15-20 minutes until golden.

5. Add your favorite pizza sauce and toppings, then return to the oven for an additional 10 minutes.

Beef and Broccoli Stir-Fry

Ingredients:

- 1 pound lean beef, thinly sliced
- 2 cups broccoli florets
- 3 cloves garlic, minced
- 1 tablespoon fresh ginger, minced
- 2 tablespoons low-sodium soy sauce
- 1 tablespoon honey or maple syrup
- 1 tablespoon sesame oil
- Salt and pepper to taste
- Cooked quinoa or brown rice for serving

Instructions:

1. In a small bowl, whisk together the soy sauce, honey or maple syrup, and sesame oil. Set aside.

2. Heat a large skillet or wok over high heat. Add a splash of oil and stir-fry the beef until browned. Remove from the skillet and set aside.

3. In the same skillet, add a bit more oil if needed, then stir-fry the garlic and ginger until fragrant.

4. Add the broccoli florets and continue to stir-fry for a few minutes until they start to soften.

5. Return the cooked beef to the skillet and pour the sauce over it. Stir-fry for another 2-3 minutes until everything is well coated and heated through.

6. Season with salt and pepper to taste. Serve over cooked quinoa or brown rice.

Pegan Spaghetti Squash Alfredo

Ingredients:

- 1 large spaghetti squash
- 1 cup unsweetened almond milk
- 1/2 cup nutritional yeast
- 2 cloves garlic, minced

- 1/2 teaspoon dried basil
- 1/2 teaspoon dried oregano
- Salt and pepper to taste
- Chopped fresh parsley for garnish

Instructions:

1. Preheat your oven to 375°F (190°C). Cut the spaghetti squash in half lengthwise, scoop out the seeds, and place the halves on a baking sheet, cut side down.
2. Bake for about 30-40 minutes or until the squash flesh can be easily shredded with a fork.
3. While the squash is baking, prepare the Alfredo sauce. In a saucepan over medium heat, combine almond milk, nutritional yeast, garlic, basil, and oregano. Stir until well combined and heated through.
4. Once the spaghetti squash is done, use a fork to shred the flesh into "noodles."
5. Pour the Alfredo sauce over the squash noodles, season with salt and pepper, and garnish with chopped fresh parsley.

Moroccan-Inspired Chickpea Stew

Ingredients:

- 2 tablespoons olive oil

- 1 onion, diced

- 2 cloves garlic, minced

- 1 tablespoon ground cumin

- 1 tablespoon ground coriander

- 1 teaspoon ground cinnamon

- 1 can (15 oz) chickpeas, drained and rinsed

- 1 can (15 oz) diced tomatoes

- 2 cups vegetable broth

- 1 cup carrots, sliced

- 1 cup sweet potatoes, diced

- 1/2 cup dried apricots, chopped

- Salt and pepper to taste

- Fresh cilantro leaves for garnish

Instructions:

1. In a large pot, heat the olive oil over medium heat. Add the diced onion and garlic and sauté until fragrant and softened.

2. Stir in the ground cumin, ground coriander, and ground cinnamon. Cook for another minute to release the spices' flavors.

3. Add the chickpeas, diced tomatoes, vegetable broth, carrots, sweet potatoes, and dried apricots to the pot.

4. Bring the stew to a boil, then reduce the heat and simmer for about 20-25 minutes or until the vegetables are tender.

5. Season with salt and pepper to taste. Garnish with fresh cilantro leaves before serving.

Stuffed Acorn Squash

Ingredients:

- 2 acorn squashes, halved and seeds removed
- 1 cup quinoa, cooked
- 1 cup black beans, cooked
- 1 cup corn kernels
- 1 red bell pepper, diced
- 1/2 cup diced red onion
- 1/2 cup fresh cilantro, chopped
- Juice of 1 lime
- 1 teaspoon ground cumin

- Salt and pepper to taste

- Avocado slices for garnish

Instructions:

1. Preheat your oven to 375°F (190°C). Place the acorn squash halves on a baking sheet, cut side down, and bake for about 30 minutes or until they are tender.

2. In a large bowl, combine cooked quinoa, black beans, corn, red bell pepper, red onion, cilantro, lime juice, ground cumin, salt, and pepper.

3. Once the squash halves are done, remove them from the oven and flip them over.

4. Stuff each squash half with the quinoa and black bean mixture.

5. Return the stuffed squash to the oven and bake for an additional 10-15 minutes until heated through.

6. Garnish with avocado slices before serving.

Lemon Herb Shrimp Skewers

Ingredients:

- 1 pound large shrimp, peeled and deveined

- Zest and juice of 2 lemons

- 2 tablespoons olive oil

- 2 cloves garlic, minced

- 1 tablespoon fresh basil, chopped

- 1 tablespoon fresh parsley, chopped

- Salt and pepper to taste

- Wooden skewers, soaked in water

Instructions:

1. In a bowl, whisk together the lemon zest, lemon juice, olive oil, minced garlic, fresh basil, fresh parsley, salt, and pepper.

2. Thread the shrimp onto the soaked wooden skewers.

3. Brush the lemon herb marinade over the shrimp skewers and let them marinate for about 15-20 minutes.

4. Preheat your grill to medium-high heat. Grill the shrimp skewers for about 2-3 minutes per side or until they turn pink and opaque.

Turkey and Sweet Potato Chili

Ingredients:

- 1 pound ground turkey

- 2 sweet potatoes, peeled and diced

- 1 onion, diced

- 2 cloves garlic, minced

- 1 can (15 oz) diced tomatoes

- 1 can (15 oz) black beans, drained and rinsed

- 2 cups vegetable broth

- 2 teaspoons chili powder

- 1 teaspoon ground cumin

- Salt and pepper to taste

- Chopped fresh cilantro for garnish

- Greek yogurt for topping (optional)

Instructions:

1. In a large pot, brown the ground turkey over medium heat. Remove the turkey from the pot and set it aside.

2. In the same pot, add a bit of olive oil if needed, then sauté the diced sweet potatoes, diced onion, and minced garlic until they begin to soften.

3. Stir in the diced tomatoes, black beans, vegetable broth, chili powder, ground cumin, salt, and pepper.

4. Return the cooked turkey to the pot and simmer the chili for about 20-25 minutes or until the sweet potatoes are tender.

5. Serve hot, garnished with chopped fresh cilantro and a dollop of Greek yogurt if desired.

Pegan Eggplant Parmesan

Ingredients:

- 2 large eggplants, sliced into rounds
- 2 cups almond flour
- 2 teaspoons dried basil
- 2 teaspoons dried oregano
- 2 cups tomato sauce (sugar-free)
- 2 cups dairy-free mozzarella cheese, shredded
- Olive oil for frying
- Fresh basil leaves for garnish

Instructions:

1. In a bowl, mix the almond flour, dried basil, and dried oregano.

2. Heat some olive oil in a skillet over medium-high heat.

3. Dredge the eggplant slices in the almond flour mixture and fry them until golden brown on both sides. Place them on paper towels to remove excess oil.

4. Preheat your oven to 350°F (175°C).

5. In a baking dish, spread a layer of tomato sauce, followed by a layer of fried eggplant slices, a sprinkle of dairy-free mozzarella cheese, and repeat until all ingredients are used.

6. Finish with a layer of sauce and mozzarella cheese on top.

7. Bake for about 20-25 minutes or until the cheese is melted and bubbly.

8. Garnish with fresh basil leaves before serving.

Ginger Tofu and Broccoli

Ingredients:

- 1 block of extra-firm tofu, cubed
- 2 cups broccoli florets
- 2 cloves garlic, minced
- 1 tablespoon fresh ginger, minced
- 2 tablespoons low-sodium soy sauce

- 1 tablespoon maple syrup

- 1 tablespoon sesame oil

- Sesame seeds for garnish

Instructions:

1. In a bowl, whisk together the soy sauce, maple syrup, and sesame oil. Set aside.

2. Heat a large skillet over medium-high heat and add a bit of oil. Stir-fry the cubed tofu until it's lightly browned on all sides. Remove it from the skillet and set aside.

3. In the same skillet, add a bit more oil if needed, then stir-fry the minced garlic and minced ginger until fragrant.

4. Add the broccoli florets and continue to stir-fry for a few minutes until they start to soften.

5. Return the cooked tofu to the skillet and pour the sauce over it. Stir-fry for another 2-3 minutes until everything is well coated and heated through.

6. Garnish with sesame seeds before serving.

Quinoa-Stuffed Bell Peppers

Ingredients:

- 4 bell peppers, any color
- 1 cup quinoa, cooked
- 1 can (15 oz) black beans, drained and rinsed
- 1 cup corn kernels
- 1 cup diced tomatoes
- 1 teaspoon chili powder
- 1/2 teaspoon ground cumin
- Salt and pepper to taste
- Chopped fresh cilantro for garnish
- Avocado slices for topping (optional)

Instructions:

1. Preheat your oven to 375°F (190°C). Cut the tops off the bell peppers and remove the seeds.
2. In a bowl, combine cooked quinoa, black beans, corn, diced tomatoes, chili powder, ground cumin, salt, and pepper.
3. Stuff each bell pepper with the quinoa mixture.

4. Place the stuffed bell peppers in a baking dish, cover
    with foil, and bake for about 25-30 minutes or until
    the peppers are tender.

5. Garnish with chopped fresh cilantro and avocado
    slices if desired.

Creamy Mushroom and Spinach Pasta

Ingredients:

- 8 oz gluten-free pasta
- 2 cups mushrooms, sliced
- 2 cups fresh spinach
- 2 cloves garlic, minced
- 1 cup unsweetened almond milk
- 1/2 cup nutritional yeast
- 1/2 teaspoon dried thyme
- Salt and pepper to taste
- Fresh parsley for garnish

Instructions:

1. Cook the gluten-free pasta according to package instructions. Drain and set aside.
2. In a large skillet, sauté the sliced mushrooms and minced garlic until the mushrooms are tender.
3. Stir in the fresh spinach and cook until wilted.
4. Pour in the unsweetened almond milk, nutritional yeast, dried thyme, salt, and pepper. Stir until well combined and heated through.
5. Add the cooked pasta to the skillet and toss to coat with the creamy mushroom and spinach sauce.
6. Garnish with fresh parsley before serving.

Teriyaki Glazed Tempeh

Ingredients:

- 1 package tempeh, cut into cubes
- 1/4 cup low-sodium soy sauce
- 2 tablespoons maple syrup
- 1 clove garlic, minced
- 1/2 teaspoon fresh ginger, minced
- 1 tablespoon sesame oil
- Sesame seeds and sliced green onions for garnish

Instructions:

1. In a bowl, whisk together the soy sauce, maple syrup, minced garlic, minced ginger, and sesame oil.

2. Marinate the tempeh cubes in the sauce for about 15-20 minutes.

3. Heat a skillet over medium-high heat and add a bit of oil. Add the marinated tempeh and cook until it's browned on all sides.

4. Pour the remaining marinade into the skillet and let it simmer for a few minutes until it thickens and coats the tempeh.

5. Garnish with sesame seeds and sliced green onions before serving.

Pesto Zoodle Bowl

Ingredients:

- 4 medium zucchinis, spiralized into noodles
- 1 cup cherry tomatoes, halved
- 1/2 cup pine nuts, toasted
- 1/2 cup fresh basil leaves
- 2 cloves garlic, minced
- 1/4 cup extra-virgin olive oil

- Juice of 1 lemon

- Salt and pepper to taste

- Grated dairy-free Parmesan cheese (optional)

Instructions:

1. In a food processor, combine fresh basil leaves, minced garlic, pine nuts, extra-virgin olive oil, lemon juice, salt, and pepper. Blend until you have a smooth pesto sauce.

2. In a large bowl, toss the zucchini noodles with the cherry tomatoes and the pesto sauce until everything is well coated.

3. Serve the zoodle mixture in bowls, garnished with additional basil leaves and grated dairy-free Parmesan cheese if desired.

Chapter 5: Snacks and Appetizers

When it comes to the Pegan diet, snacks and appetizers can be just as satisfying and nutritious as your main meals. These delicious bites are perfect for satisfying your cravings while staying true to your Pegan lifestyle. Let's dive into these delectable recipes that will keep you energized throughout the day.

Guacamole with Veggie Sticks

Ingredients:

- 2 ripe avocados
- 1 small red onion, finely chopped
- 2 cloves garlic, minced
- 2 ripe tomatoes, diced
- 1 lime, juiced
- Salt and pepper to taste
- Assorted veggie sticks (carrots, cucumber, bell peppers) for dipping

Instructions:

1. Cut the avocados in half, remove the pits, and scoop the flesh into a bowl.

2. Mash the avocados with a fork.

3. Stir in the red onion, garlic, tomatoes, and lime juice.

4. Season with salt and pepper to taste.

5. Serve the guacamole with a colorful array of veggie sticks for dipping.

Roasted Red Pepper Hummus

Ingredients:

- 1 can (15 oz) chickpeas, drained and rinsed
- 2 roasted red peppers, peeled and chopped
- 2 cloves garlic, minced
- 3 tablespoons tahini
- 3 tablespoons lemon juice
- 2 tablespoons olive oil
- 1/2 teaspoon cumin
- Salt and pepper to taste

Instructions:

1. In a food processor, combine chickpeas, roasted red peppers, garlic, tahini, lemon juice, olive oil, and cumin.
2. Blend until smooth, scraping down the sides as needed.
3. Season with salt and pepper to taste.
4. Serve with fresh veggies or whole-grain crackers.

Pegan Trail Mix

Ingredients:

- 1 cup raw almonds
- 1 cup raw cashews
- 1/2 cup unsweetened coconut flakes
- 1/2 cup dried cranberries
- 1/4 cup dark chocolate chips (70% cocoa or higher)

Instructions:

1. In a large bowl, combine almonds, cashews, coconut flakes, dried cranberries, and dark chocolate chips.
2. Toss to mix well.

3. Portion into snack-sized bags for easy, on-the-go munching.

Cucumber and Tomato Salsa

Ingredients:

- 2 cucumbers, diced
- 2 ripe tomatoes, diced
- 1 red onion, finely chopped
- 1/4 cup fresh cilantro, chopped
- 1 jalapeño pepper, seeded and minced
- Juice of 2 limes
- Salt and pepper to taste

Instructions:

1. In a bowl, combine diced cucumbers, tomatoes, red onion, cilantro, and jalapeño.
2. Squeeze lime juice over the mixture and toss gently.
3. Season with salt and pepper to taste.
4. Serve as a refreshing salsa with whole-grain tortilla chips or veggie slices.

Spicy Edamame

Ingredients:

- 2 cups edamame (young soybeans), cooked and shelled
- 1 tablespoon olive oil
- 1 teaspoon chili powder
- 1/2 teaspoon paprika
- 1/4 teaspoon cayenne pepper (adjust to your spice preference)
- Salt to taste

Instructions:

1. In a bowl, toss cooked edamame with olive oil, chili powder, paprika, and cayenne pepper.
2. Sprinkle with salt and toss to coat evenly.
3. Spread the seasoned edamame on a baking sheet and bake at 375°F (190°C) for about 15 minutes until they become slightly crispy.
4. Allow them to cool slightly before serving.

Almond-Stuffed Dates

Ingredients:

- 15 Medjool dates, pitted
- 30 whole almonds (2 per date)
- A pinch of sea salt

Instructions:

1. Carefully slit open each Medjool date and remove the pit.
2. Stuff each date with two whole almonds.
3. Sprinkle a pinch of sea salt over the stuffed dates.
4. Arrange them on a platter for a sweet and nutty snack.

Stuffed Mini Peppers

Ingredients:

- 15 mini bell peppers
- 1 cup hummus (store-bought or homemade)
- Fresh herbs for garnish (e.g., parsley or chives)

Instructions:

1. Cut the tops off the mini bell peppers and remove the seeds.

2. Fill each pepper with a spoonful of hummus.

3. Garnish with fresh herbs for a burst of flavor.

4. Arrange them on a plate for a colorful and tasty appetizer.

Coconut-Crusted Tofu Bites

Ingredients:

- 1 block of firm tofu, cut into bite-sized cubes
- 1/2 cup unsweetened shredded coconut
- 2 tablespoons coconut flour
- 1/2 teaspoon garlic powder
- 1/2 teaspoon paprika
- Salt and pepper to taste
- 2 tablespoons coconut oil for frying

Instructions:

1. In a bowl, combine shredded coconut, coconut flour, garlic powder, paprika, salt, and pepper.

2. Coat each tofu cube in the coconut mixture, pressing gently to adhere.

3. Heat coconut oil in a skillet over medium heat.

4. Fry the coated tofu cubes until they turn golden brown and crispy.

5. Serve with a dipping sauce of your choice.

Greek Yogurt Dip with Veggies

Ingredients:

- 1 cup Greek yogurt
- 1 tablespoon fresh dill, chopped
- 1 tablespoon fresh mint, chopped
- 1 clove garlic, minced
- 1 cucumber, diced
- Salt and pepper to taste

Instructions:

1. In a bowl, combine Greek yogurt, fresh dill, fresh mint, and minced garlic.

2. Season with salt and pepper to taste.

3. Serve the creamy dip with an assortment of fresh veggies for dipping.

Avocado and Cilantro Lime Dip

Ingredients:

- 2 ripe avocados
- 1/4 cup fresh cilantro, chopped
- Juice of 2 limes
- 1 clove garlic, minced
- Salt and pepper to taste

Instructions:

1. Scoop the flesh of the ripe avocados into a bowl.
2. Mash the avocados with a fork.
3. Stir in fresh cilantro, lime juice, minced garlic, salt, and pepper.
4. Serve this zesty dip with veggie sticks or whole-grain crackers.

Zucchini Fritters

Ingredients:

- 2 zucchinis, grated
- 1/4 cup almond flour
- 2 eggs

- 1/4 cup fresh basil, chopped
- 1/4 cup fresh parsley, chopped
- Salt and pepper to taste
- Olive oil for frying

Instructions:

1. Place grated zucchini in a clean kitchen towel and squeeze out excess moisture.
2. In a bowl, combine grated zucchini, almond flour, eggs, fresh basil, fresh parsley, salt, and pepper.
3. Heat olive oil in a skillet over medium-high heat.
4. Spoon portions of the zucchini mixture into the skillet and flatten to make fritters.
5. Cook until golden brown on both sides.
6. Serve these crispy fritters hot.

Roasted Chickpeas

Ingredients:

- 2 cans (15 oz each) chickpeas, drained and rinsed
- 2 tablespoons olive oil
- 1 teaspoon smoked paprika

- 1/2 teaspoon cayenne pepper (adjust to your spice preference)
- Salt and pepper to taste

Instructions:

1. Preheat your oven to 400°F (200°C).
2. In a bowl, toss chickpeas with olive oil, smoked paprika, cayenne pepper, salt, and pepper.
3. Spread the seasoned chickpeas on a baking sheet and roast for about 30-40 minutes, or until they are crispy and golden.
4. Let them cool before munching on these crunchy, protein-packed snacks.

Mixed Nut Energy Bars

Ingredients:

- 1 cup mixed nuts (almonds, cashews, walnuts), chopped
- 1 cup dates, pitted and chopped
- 1/4 cup unsweetened shredded coconut
- 2 tablespoons almond butter
- 1/4 cup dried cranberries

- 1/4 cup dark chocolate chips (70% cocoa or higher)

Instructions:

1. In a food processor, combine chopped mixed nuts, dates, shredded coconut, almond butter, and dried cranberries.
2. Pulse until the mixture sticks together.
3. Press the mixture into a square baking dish and sprinkle dark chocolate chips on top, pressing them in gently.
4. Refrigerate until firm, then cut into bars for a satisfying, on-the-go snack.

Pegan Popcorn

Ingredients:

- 1/2 cup popcorn kernels
- 2 tablespoons coconut oil
- Nutritional yeast for seasoning (optional)
- Salt to taste

Instructions:

1. Heat coconut oil in a large pot with a lid over medium-high heat.
2. Add popcorn kernels, cover with the lid, and shake the pot occasionally until the popping slows down.
3. Remove from heat, and while the popcorn is hot, season with nutritional yeast (for a cheesy flavor) and salt to taste.
4. Toss to evenly distribute the seasonings.

Sweet Potato Fries with Chipotle Aioli

Ingredients for Fries:

- 2 sweet potatoes, cut into fries
- 2 tablespoons olive oil
- 1 teaspoon paprika
- 1/2 teaspoon garlic powder
- Salt and pepper to taste

Ingredients for Chipotle Aioli:

- 1/2 cup mayonnaise (or vegan mayo)

- 1 chipotle pepper in adobo sauce, minced

- 1 clove garlic, minced

- 1 tablespoon lime juice

- Salt and pepper to taste

Instructions for Fries:

1. Preheat your oven to 425°F (220°C).

2. In a bowl, toss sweet potato fries with olive oil, paprika, garlic powder, salt, and pepper.

3. Spread the fries on a baking sheet and roast for 20-25 minutes, flipping halfway through, until they are crispy.

Instructions for Chipotle Aioli:

1. In a small bowl, mix together mayonnaise, minced chipotle pepper, minced garlic, lime juice, salt, and pepper.

2. Serve the sweet potato fries with a side of chipotle aioli for dipping.

Chapter 6: Desserts

Indulge in the delightful world of Pegan desserts! These sweet creations not only satisfy your cravings but also align with the Pegan lifestyle. From creamy mousse to fruity parfaits, we've got you covered with a range of delicious options. Let's dive into these delectable dessert recipes.

Pegan Chocolate Avocado Mousse

Ingredients:

- 2 ripe avocados
- 1/4 cup unsweetened cocoa powder
- 1/4 cup maple syrup
- 1 tsp vanilla extract
- Pinch of salt

Instructions:

1. Blend avocados, cocoa powder, maple syrup, vanilla extract, and a pinch of salt until smooth.
2. Chill in the refrigerator for at least 30 minutes.
3. Serve with a sprinkle of shaved dark chocolate.

Mixed Berry Chia Seed Pudding

Ingredients:

- 1/2 cup mixed berries (strawberries, blueberries, raspberries)
- 2 tbsp chia seeds
- 1 cup almond milk
- 1 tsp honey (optional)

Instructions:

1. Mash the mixed berries and mix them with chia seeds, almond milk, and honey (if desired).
2. Refrigerate for a few hours or overnight until it thickens.
3. Top with additional berries before serving.

Almond Butter Cups

Ingredients:

- 1/2 cup almond butter
- 1/4 cup coconut oil
- 2 tbsp cocoa powder
- 2 tbsp maple syrup

Instructions:

1. Melt coconut oil and mix it with almond butter, cocoa powder, and maple syrup.

2. Pour the mixture into silicone molds or mini muffin cups.

3. Freeze until firm and enjoy!

Coconut Macaroons

Ingredients:

- 2 cups shredded coconut
- 1/2 cup almond flour
- 1/4 cup maple syrup
- 1/4 cup coconut oil
- 1 tsp vanilla extract

Instructions:

1. Combine shredded coconut and almond flour in a bowl.

2. Mix in maple syrup, melted coconut oil, and vanilla extract.

3. Form into macaroon shapes and bake at 325°F (163°C) for 15-20 minutes or until golden.

Pegan Banana Bread

Ingredients:

- 3 ripe bananas
- 1/2 cup almond flour
- 1/4 cup coconut flour
- 3 eggs
- 1/4 cup maple syrup
- 1 tsp baking soda

Instructions:

1. Mash bananas and mix with almond flour, coconut flour, eggs, maple syrup, and baking soda.
2. Pour into a loaf pan and bake at 350°F (175°C) for 45-50 minutes.

Chocolate Dipped Strawberries

Ingredients:

- 12 fresh strawberries
- 1/4 cup dark chocolate chips
- 1 tsp coconut oil

- Toppings (chopped nuts, shredded coconut, or sea salt)

Instructions:

1. Melt dark chocolate chips with coconut oil in a microwave or using a double boiler.
2. Dip each strawberry into the melted chocolate, coating it partially.
3. Place on parchment paper and sprinkle with your choice of toppings.
4. Allow to cool and harden in the refrigerator before serving.

Blueberry Almond Crisp

Ingredients:

- 2 cups fresh blueberries
- 1/2 cup almond flour
- 1/4 cup coconut oil
- 1/4 cup maple syrup
- 1/2 cup sliced almonds

Instructions:

1. Toss blueberries in a baking dish.

2. In a bowl, mix almond flour, melted coconut oil, and maple syrup.

3. Sprinkle the almond mixture over the blueberries.

4. Top with sliced almonds and bake at 350°F (175°C) for 25-30 minutes or until golden and bubbly.

Pecan Pie Energy Bites

Ingredients:

- 1 cup pecans
- 1/2 cup dates (soaked and pitted)
- 1/4 cup shredded coconut
- 1 tsp vanilla extract
- Pinch of salt

Instructions:

1. Blend pecans, soaked dates, shredded coconut, vanilla extract, and a pinch of salt in a food processor until a dough forms.

2. Roll into bite-sized balls and refrigerate until firm.

No-Bake Cashew Cheesecake

Ingredients:

- 1 1/2 cups cashews (soaked and drained)
- 1/4 cup coconut oil
- 1/4 cup maple syrup
- 1 tsp vanilla extract
- Juice of 1 lemon
- Pinch of salt

Instructions:

1. Blend soaked cashews, melted coconut oil, maple syrup, vanilla extract, lemon juice, and a pinch of salt until creamy.
2. Pour into a pie crust or a silicone mold.
3. Chill in the refrigerator until set.

Avocado Chocolate Truffles

Ingredients:

- 2 ripe avocados
- 1/4 cup cocoa powder
- 1/4 cup coconut flour

- 1/4 cup maple syrup

- 1 tsp vanilla extract

Instructions:

1. Mash avocados and mix with cocoa powder, coconut flour, maple syrup, and vanilla extract.
2. Roll into truffle-sized balls and refrigerate until firm.

Lemon Poppy Seed Muffins

Ingredients:

- 1 1/2 cups almond flour
- 1/4 cup coconut flour
- 1/4 cup maple syrup
- Zest and juice of 2 lemons
- 3 eggs
- 1 tsp baking soda
- 1 tbsp poppy seeds

Instructions:

1. Mix almond flour, coconut flour, maple syrup, lemon zest, lemon juice, eggs, baking soda, and poppy seeds until well combined.

2. Spoon the batter into muffin cups and bake at 350°F (175°C) for 20-25 minutes.

Raspberry Coconut Bars

Ingredients:

- 2 cups raspberries (fresh or frozen)
- 1 cup shredded coconut
- 1/4 cup coconut oil
- 1/4 cup maple syrup
- 1 tsp vanilla extract

Instructions:

1. Combine raspberries, shredded coconut, melted coconut oil, maple syrup, and vanilla extract in a bowl.
2. Press the mixture into a baking dish and refrigerate until set.
3. Cut into bars and serve.

Apple Cinnamon Oat Cookies

Ingredients:

- 2 cups rolled oats
- 1 cup applesauce
- 1/4 cup almond butter
- 1/4 cup maple syrup
- 1 tsp cinnamon
- 1/2 cup diced apples

Instructions:

1. Mix rolled oats, applesauce, almond butter, maple syrup, cinnamon, and diced apples in a bowl.
2. Drop spoonfuls of the dough onto a baking sheet and bake at 350°F (175°C) for 12-15 minutes.

Mango Sorbet

Ingredients:

- 2 ripe mangoes (peeled and diced)
- 1/4 cup coconut milk
- 2 tbsp honey (optional)

Instructions:

1. Blend ripe mangoes, coconut milk, and honey (if desired) until smooth.

2. Pour into a container and freeze until firm, stirring occasionally.

Pegan Berry Parfait

Ingredients:

- 1 cup mixed berries (strawberries, blueberries, raspberries)
- 1/2 cup coconut yogurt
- 1/4 cup granola (Pegan-friendly)
- 1 tsp honey (optional)

Instructions:

1. Layer mixed berries, coconut yogurt, and granola in a glass or jar.

2. Drizzle with honey if desired.

3. Repeat the layers and serve chilled.

In this chapter, we've curated a delightful collection of smoothie recipes that are not only delicious but also packed with the goodness of the Pegan diet. Each smoothie is carefully crafted to provide a burst of flavors and nutrients to keep you energized and satisfied.

Green Goddess Smoothie

Ingredients:

- 1 cup fresh spinach leaves
- 1/2 cucumber, peeled and chopped
- 1 green apple, cored and sliced
- 1/2 lemon, juiced
- 1/2 cup coconut water
- Ice cubes (optional)

Instructions:

1. Place all the ingredients in a blender.
2. Blend until smooth and creamy.
3. Add ice cubes if desired, and blend again.

4. Pour into a glass and enjoy your refreshing Green Goddess Smoothie!

Berry Blast Smoothie

Ingredients:

- 1 cup mixed berries (strawberries, blueberries, raspberries)
- 1/2 banana
- 1/2 cup almond milk
- 1 tablespoon chia seeds
- Honey or maple syrup for sweetness (optional)

Instructions:

1. Combine the berries, banana, almond milk, and chia seeds in a blender.
2. Blend until the mixture is smooth.
3. Add honey or maple syrup if you prefer it sweeter.
4. Pour into a glass and savor the Berry Blast Smoothie.

Tropical Paradise Smoothie

Ingredients:

- 1 cup frozen tropical fruit blend (mango, pineapple, papaya)
- 1/2 cup coconut milk
- 1/2 cup Greek yogurt
- 1 tablespoon honey (optional)

Instructions:

1. Add the frozen tropical fruit, coconut milk, Greek yogurt, and honey (if desired) to a blender.
2. Blend until silky smooth.
3. Pour into a glass, close your eyes, and transport yourself to a Tropical Paradise!

Peanut Butter Banana Smoothie

Ingredients:

- 1 banana
- 2 tablespoons natural peanut butter
- 1 cup almond milk
- 1 tablespoon flaxseeds

- 1/2 teaspoon cinnamon

- Ice cubes (optional)

Instructions:

1. Place the banana, peanut butter, almond milk, flaxseeds, and cinnamon in a blender.
2. Blend until creamy.
3. Add ice cubes for a colder, thicker consistency.
4. Pour into a glass and indulge in the Peanut Butter Banana Smoothie.

Chocolate Protein Smoothie

Ingredients:

- 1 scoop chocolate protein powder
- 1 cup unsweetened almond milk
- 1 tablespoon cocoa powder
- 1/2 banana
- 1 tablespoon almond butter
- Ice cubes (optional)

Instructions:

1. Combine the chocolate protein powder, almond milk, cocoa powder, banana, and almond butter in a blender.

2. Blend until you have a rich, chocolatey concoction.

3. If you like it colder, add ice cubes and blend again.

4. Pour into a glass and relish the Chocolate Protein Smoothie.

Spinach and Pineapple Smoothie

Ingredients:

*   2 cups fresh spinach leaves
*   1 cup pineapple chunks
*   1/2 cup coconut water
*   1/2 lime, juiced
*   1 tablespoon honey (optional)

Instructions:

1. Add spinach, pineapple chunks, coconut water, lime juice, and honey (if desired) to the blender.

2. Blend until you achieve a vibrant green mixture.

3. Pour into a glass and enjoy the nutritious Spinach and Pineapple Smoothie.

Mango Coconut Smoothie

Ingredients:

- 1 cup ripe mango chunks
- 1/2 cup coconut milk
- 1/2 cup Greek yogurt
- 1 tablespoon shredded coconut
- Ice cubes (optional)

Instructions:

1. Combine mango chunks, coconut milk, Greek yogurt, and shredded coconut in a blender.
2. Blend until it's thick and tropical.
3. If you like it frosty, toss in some ice cubes and blend again.
4. Pour into a glass and savor the Mango Coconut Smoothie.

Blueberry Almond Smoothie

Ingredients:

- 1 cup blueberries
- 1/2 cup unsweetened almond milk
- 1/4 cup almonds
- 1/2 teaspoon vanilla extract
- Honey or maple syrup for sweetness (optional)

Instructions:

1. Add blueberries, almond milk, almonds, and vanilla extract to the blender.
2. Blend until smooth and creamy.
3. Add honey or maple syrup for a touch of sweetness if desired.
4. Pour into a glass and relish the Blueberry Almond Smoothie.

Kale and Kiwi Smoothie

Ingredients:

- 1 cup kale leaves, stems removed
- 2 kiwis, peeled and sliced

- 1/2 lime, juiced
- 1 tablespoon honey (optional)
- 1 cup water or coconut water

Instructions:

1. Place kale, kiwis, lime juice, honey (if desired), and water or coconut water in a blender.
2. Blend until the kale is well incorporated and the smoothie is green and vibrant.
3. Pour into a glass and enjoy the nutritious Kale and Kiwi Smoothie.

Avocado Power Smoothie

Ingredients:

- 1 ripe avocado
- 1 cup spinach leaves
- 1/2 banana
- 1 tablespoon chia seeds
- 1 cup almond milk
- Ice cubes (optional)

Instructions:

1. Combine the ripe avocado, spinach leaves, banana, chia seeds, almond milk, and ice cubes (if desired) in a blender.

2. Blend until you have a creamy, green delight.

3. Pour into a glass and experience the Avocado Power Smoothie.

Cucumber Mint Smoothie

Ingredients:

- 1 cucumber, peeled and chopped
- 1/4 cup fresh mint leaves
- 1/2 lime, juiced
- 1 cup coconut water
- 1 tablespoon honey (optional)

Instructions:

1. Add cucumber, fresh mint leaves, lime juice, coconut water, and honey (if desired) to the blender.

2. Blend until the mixture is smooth and refreshing.

3. Pour into a glass and savor the cool Cucumber Mint Smoothie.

Pegan Pumpkin Spice Smoothie

Ingredients:

- 1/2 cup canned pumpkin puree
- 1/2 banana
- 1 teaspoon pumpkin spice blend
- 1 cup almond milk
- 1 tablespoon maple syrup

Instructions:

1. Combine pumpkin puree, banana, pumpkin spice blend, almond milk, and maple syrup in a blender.
2. Blend until smooth and creamy with a delightful pumpkin spice aroma.
3. Pour into a glass and embrace the flavors of fall with the Pegan Pumpkin Spice Smoothie.

Peach and Oat Smoothie

Ingredients:

- 1 cup ripe peaches, sliced
- 1/2 cup rolled oats
- 1/2 cup almond milk

- 1 tablespoon honey (optional)
- 1/2 teaspoon vanilla extract

Instructions:

1. Combine ripe peaches, rolled oats, almond milk, honey (if desired), and vanilla extract in a blender.
2. Blend until you have a creamy and satisfying Peach and Oat Smoothie.
3. Pour into a glass and enjoy this wholesome treat.

Berry Spinach Smoothie

Ingredients:

- 1 cup fresh spinach leaves
- 1/2 cup mixed berries (strawberries, blueberries, raspberries)
- 1/2 banana
- 1 cup almond milk
- 1 tablespoon chia seeds

Instructions:

1. Add fresh spinach leaves, mixed berries, banana, almond milk, and chia seeds to the blender.

2. Blend until the smoothie turns a beautiful shade of purple.

3. Pour into a glass and savor the Berry Spinach Smoothie, packed with antioxidants.

Chocolate Avocado Smoothie

Ingredients:

- 1 ripe avocado
- 2 tablespoons cocoa powder
- 1 cup almond milk
- 1 tablespoon honey or maple syrup
- Ice cubes (optional)

Instructions:

1. Place the ripe avocado, cocoa powder, almond milk, honey or maple syrup, and ice cubes (if desired) in a blender.

2. Blend until you have a creamy, chocolate-infused concoction.

3. Pour into a glass and treat yourself to the indulgent Chocolate Avocado Smoothie.

CONCLUSION

As we reach the final chapter of this cookbook, it's not just an ending but the beginning of a new chapter in your culinary journey. The "Pegan Diet Cookbook" has guided you through a diverse array of recipes, helping you discover the delicious fusion of paleo and vegan principles. But now, let's reflect on what this journey has meant and where it can take you.

This conclusion is not about bidding farewell to your Pegan experience; rather, it's about embracing it as a lifestyle. The recipes you've explored in this book are just the tip of the iceberg. They've introduced you to a world of flavors and ingredients that can transform the way you eat, think about food, and nourish your body.

Staying Pegan for Life:

- **Sustainability**: The Pegan diet isn't a short-term fix; it's a sustainable way of eating that can benefit your health for years to come. Consider how you can incorporate Pegan principles into your daily meals and make it a lifelong commitment.

- **Flexibility**: Remember that the Pegan diet is flexible and adaptable. Feel free to tweak recipes, experiment with new ingredients, and make it your own. This flexibility ensures that your Pegan journey remains exciting and tailored to your tastes.

- **Community**: Joining a Pegan community can be incredibly motivating. Share your experiences, swap tips, and connect with others who are on a similar path. Building a support network can help you stay committed and inspired.

- **Mindful Eating**: Take a moment to appreciate the connection between what you eat and how it makes you feel. Practice mindful eating, savoring each bite, and paying attention to your body's signals of hunger and fullness.

In summary, the "Pegan Diet Cookbook" is not just a book; it's a gateway to a healthier, more conscious way of eating. As you move forward, continue to explore, experiment, and enjoy the culinary adventure that the Pegan diet offers. May your Pegan journey be filled with delicious discoveries and vibrant health.

www.ingramcontent.com/pod-product-compliance
Lightning Source LLC
Chambersburg PA
CBHW070901260726
48661CB00004B/1524